Bodybuilding Programming and Training

Build your workout

©2021 Andrea Raimondi
www.fitnessedintorni.it

AREdit.com

[3]

To Luciano e Pinuccia

INDEX

=== Andrea Raimondi ===

Introduction

Sometimes, in the gym, I hear speeches related to training full of irrationality and nonsense.

Sometimes it happens to hear people who maybe have been training for years and still don't know what they are doing.

They don't know why they perform 5 or 10 repetitions, why they do 3 sets and not 5. Or they load weight randomly.

Sometimes it happens to see personal trainers who perform exercises with bad executions: too fast, with a rebound, or they help to lift the bar to close a last "fundamental" repetition.

This book was written with those people in mind, knowing that they will never read it.

This book will be read by those who want to understand what they have been told to do in the gym.

This book will be read by those who want to be independent and want to be able to create their personalized training.

This book will be read by those who want to acquire solid foundations relating to programming and the construction of training workouts.

If you need advice on the construction of your training plans, mesocycles, or macrocycles, you can write to me at info@fitnessedintorni.it.

Periodization

Periodizing means **planning** a training program to correctly manage the training variables to ensure an optimal response from the body concerning the goal you want to achieve, whether it is the increase in muscle mass or strength.

Based on the **general adaptation syndrome theory**, it is assumed that the body subjected to the stress of exercise reacts by increasing protein synthesis and other metabolic mechanisms that lead to the over-compensation of the muscles proteins, thus initiating the process of increasing and strengthening the capabilities of the muscles themselves.

But over time, the muscle, if subjected to the same stimulus, slows down or stops growth precisely due to the body's ability to adapt. Hence the need to vary the training stimuli by altering the training variables to ensure the desired compensatory response.

Periodizing also means inserting the single training session within a cycle of sessions.

Usually, we speak of **macrocycle**, **mesocycle**, **microcycle**.

The *microcycle* can be considered the single week of training sessions, the *mesocycle* groups a series of microcycles. A set of mesocycles constitutes the *macrocycle*.

The art of bodybuilding and body recomposition essentially consists of planning (and executing!) micro, meso, and macrocycle so that it is functional to the acquisition of muscle mass, obviously without forgetting the role of proper nutrition.

It is clear that the optimal solution is to find a training plan tailored to each individual. Proper planning will prevent the body from getting used to training stress because it is able to make changes in the main training variables, as mentioned earlier: intensity, volume, rest intervals, frequency, exercise selection, effort required.

Three types of periodization can be identified: **traditional linear** periodization, non-linear or **wavy** periodization, **inverse** periodization.

In traditional periodization, there is an inverse relationship between volume and intensity. This leads to alternating high volume and low-intensity mesocycles with low volume and high-intensity mesocycles (load). We then pass from a period of high volumes to one of low volumes by increasing the intensity. This can lead to an increase in metabolic stress and lead in some cases (but this ultimately applies to the high-level athlete) to the threshold of overtraining.

To overcome the problems of metabolic stress induced by traditional periodization and to maintain a greater hypertrophic state (the volume, as we know, is one of the factors of hypertrophy), several changes have been proposed to the traditional approach.

Some of these approaches propose varying volume and intensity within the same mesocycle, alternating high-volume weeks with high-intensity weeks, creating a wavy periodization.

The inverse periodization leads to insert a period of hypertrophy, increasing the volume and reducing the load, at the end of a traditional macrocycle.

At present, however, there is no scientific evidence on which is the best approach for hypertrophy. Moreover, the hypertrophic response ultimately depends on the individual response to the set of factors that govern the hypertrophy itself: it will never be possible to reproduce the same conditions on the single individual who once follows the traditional periodization approach and another time the wave periodization approach.

Ultimately, the individual response given by one's genetics counts, all other conditions being equal. How many muscle fibers of type I and type II an individual have in his muscles. Someone will get more muscle development from high volume and low intensity, others from high intensity and low volume.

The magic and skill of the trainer consists in using and manipulating the training variables to find the best solution for the individual, ensuring a condition that does not reach overtraining.

In general we can for convenience keep in mind the following values to create our workout plans.

Metabolic phase
Sets: 2/3
Reps: 20/25
Load up to 60% 1RM

Hypertrophy phase
Sets: 3/4
Reps: 6/12
Load at 60% -80% 1RM

Strength phase
Sets: 4/5
Reps: 3/5
Load at 85% -100% 1RM

We can build on these parameters the periodization of the mesocycles or microcycles by varying volume, load, increasing or decreasing the recovery between the sets, alternating the execution speed, always with the correct movement.

TRAINING FREQUENCY

We can decide within the mesocycle to adopt **full-body** strategies or strategies based on **split routines**.

With full-body training, all major muscle groups are trained in each session.

With split routines, on the other hand, it is decided to train only a few muscle groups in each session.

The choice depends on the time available and the individual's training skills. All these techniques aim to train all the muscle groups more than once in the microcycle, which usually corresponds to a week.

There is not much to argue about full-body training, in any case when training all the muscles there are no particular strategies other than the choice of the exercise to be performed.

Usually, full-body workouts do not guarantee adequate recovery to the muscles. For this reason some systems have been developed over time that allows an increase in the training frequency, allowing adequate recovery to the trained muscles at the same time. All this is achieved by using split routines during the microcycle (usually the week) of training.

A split routine consists simply of dividing the muscles over the different training days, usually four days per week at least.

In the following pages, I have included the main types of split routines.

EXAMPLE of Full-Body Workout

Session	Exercise	Volume
Back, Shoulders, Chest Biceps, Triceps Quadriceps, hamstrings Glutes, Abdominals	Bench press	3 x 10
	Pulley	3 x 10
	Pull down	3 x 10
	Military Press	4 x 10
	Dumbbells Curl	3 x 10
	Leg Curl	3 x 15
	Squat	3 x 10
	Leg Extension	3 x 15
	Calf	4 x 12
	Crunch	3 x 30

Split Upper/Lower Body

This split involves training the upper body in one session and the lower body in another. Usually from one to three exercises are used for each muscle district, with a frequency of at least four weekly sessions (two for the upper body and two for the lower body).

EXAMPLE of Upper Body / Lower Body Split Routine

Session	Exercise	Volume
A **Upper Body** Back, Shoulders, Chest Biceps, Triceps	Pull-ups	3 x Max
	Dumbbell Row	3 x 10
	Dumbbells Curl	3 x 10
	French Press	3 x 10
	Military Press	4 x 10
	Bench Press	3 x 10
	Inclinded Bench Press	3 x 10
B **Upper Body** Quadriceps, Hamstrings Glutes, Abdominals	Leg Curl	3 x 15
	Leg Press	3 x 20
	Leg Extension	3 x 15
	Calf	4 x 12
	Lunge	3 x 10
	Crunch	3 x 30

Push / Pull Routine

With this type of routine, the muscles are divided according to the type of movement, that is, between muscles that serve to push and muscles that serve to pull. Session A is for pushing muscles and session B is for traction muscles. Four sessions per week. If there are three weekly sessions planned, it is possible to alternate between one week and another: A-B-A the initial week and B-A-B the following week, and so on.
Depending on the time available, it is possible to insert more than one exercise per muscle group.

EXAMPLE of Push / Pull Routine

Session	Exercise	Volume
A **Push** Shoulders, Chest, Triceps, Quadriceps, Abs	Military Press	4 x 10
	Squat	3 x 10
	Crunch	3 x 30
	French Press	3 x 10
	Bench Press	3 x 10
B **Pull** Dorsal, Femoral Biceps, Low back	Curl Dumbbells	3 x 10
	Chin-up	3 x max
	Leg Curl	3 x 15
	Deadlift	3 x 12

Planes of motion Split

This split routine involves dividing the training sessions according to the planes of movement: vertical and horizontal pushing movements, vertical and horizontal pulling movements. For the legs, there are predominant exercises for the quadriceps or the hips.

One training session will be dedicated to vertical movement exercises and another to horizontal movement exercises, including exercises for the predominant quadriceps legs or, alternatively, exercises with predominant movement at the hip level. Two to four weekly sessions are planned.

EXAMPLE di Planes of motion Split

Session	Exercise	Volume
A Horizontal Plane Movements Quad dominant Legs movements	Leg Extension	3 x 15
	Squat	3 x 10
	Bench Press	3 x 10
	Dumbbell lateral raise	3 x 10
	Curl dumbbells	4 x 10
	Crunch	3 x 30
B Vertical Plane Movements Hip dominant Legs movements	Leg Curl	3 x 15
	Chin-ups	4 x max
	Military Press	3 x 12
	Pull Down Rope	3 x 12
	French Press	3 x 10
	Crunch	3 x 30

Push, Pull, Legs and complementary exercise

In this split routine model, each session is made of "**basic**" exercises for legs, push movements, pull movements and a **complementary** exercise, alternating between the three movements.
Two to five sessions per week, alternating the exercises from week to week

EXAMPLE Push, Pull, Legs and complementary exercise

Session	Type	Exercise	Volume
A	**Push Basic** Choose an exercise	Bench Press	3 x 15
		Inclinded bench press	3 x 10
		Dip	3 x 10
		Military Press	3 x 10
	Push Complementary Choose an exercise	Dumbbells bench press	4 x 10
		Cable crossover	3 x 12
	Pull Basic Choose an exercise	Chin up	3 x max
		Barbell Row	3 x 12
		Dumbbell Row	3 x 12
	Leg Basic Choose an exercise	Squat	3 x 10
		DeadLift	3 x 10

Session	Type	Exercise	Volume
B	**Push Basic** Choose an exercise	Bench Press	3 x 15
		Inclined Bench Press	3 x 10
		Dip	3 x 10
		Military Press	3 x 10
	Pull Basic Choose an exercise	Pull Up	3 x max
		Barbell Row	3 x 12
		Dumbbell Row	3 x 12
	Pull Complementary Choose an exercise	Pulley	3 x 12
		Lat machine	3 x 12
		Dumbbell lateral raise	3 x 12
	Leg Basic Choose an exercise	Squat	3 x 10
		DeadLift	3 x 10

Session	Type	Exercise	Volume
C	**Push Basic** Choose an exercise	Bench Press	3 x 15
		Inclined Bench Press	3 x 10
		Dip	3 x 10
		Military Press	3 x 10
	Pull Basic Choose an exercise	Pull Up	3 x max
		Barbell Row	3 x 12
		Dumbbell Row	3 x 12
	Leg Basic Choose an exercise	Squat	3 x 10
		DeadLift	3 x 10
	Leg Complementary Choose an exercise	Lunge	3 x 12
		Leg Press	3 x 12
		Leg extension	3 x 12

Russian Split Routine

It is a split routine used a lot in Powerlifting, it includes at least three weekly sessions in which a muscle group between legs, chest and back is highlighted in a given session, adding complementary and/or exercises for the arms. In Powerlifting the so-called "fundamental" exercises are clearly privileged: squat, bench press, deadlift.

EXAMPLE Russian Split Routine

Session	Exercise	Volume
A **Legs** **Chest**	Squat	4 x 8
	Bench Press	3 x 10
	Leg Press	3 x 12
	Lunge	3 x 12
B **Chest** **Legs** **Triceps**	Bench Press	4 x 10
	Squat	3 x 10
	Inclined Dumbbells Bench Press	3 x 12
	French Press	3 x 12
C **Dorsal,** **Biceps**	DeadLift	4 x 8
	Dumbbell Row	3 x 10
	Pulley	3 x 12
	Dumbbell Curl	3 x 10

Split "Raimondi"

This is the routine that I usually propose to those who train with me. It consists of five weekly sessions in which to alternate the sessions as follows A-B-C-A-B. The lacking muscles are trained at least three times a week while the other muscle groups at least twice. In the example below, you will find a routine that assumes that legs are muscles to train more.

EXAMPLE Split "Raimondi"

Session	Exercise	Volume
A **Legs** **Chest**	Leg Curl	4 x 12
	Bench Press	4 x 12
	Leg Extension	4 x 12
	Dumbbells flyes	4 x 12
B **Back** **Shoulders**	Military Press	4 x 12
	Dumbbell lateral raise	4 x 12
	Pulley	4 x 12
	Lat machine	4 x 12
C **Legs,** **Biceps,** **Triceps**	Pull Down Corda	4 x 12
	Dumbbells curl	4 x 12
	Leg Extension	4 x 12
	Leg Press	4 x 12

EXAMPLES OF PERIODIZATION

An example of ***traditional periodization*** can consist of the following mesocycles:

4 weeks of full-body *general conditioning* with three sessions per week

4 weeks of full body *hypertrophy* with three sessions per week

4 weeks of full-body *strength* with three sessions per week

WEEKS	1	2	3	4	5	6	7	8	9	10	11	12
Fase metabolica	■	■	■	■								
Fase ipertrofia					■	■	■	■				
Fase forza									■	■	■	■

An example of ***wavy periodization*** can be the following:

3 weeks of full-body *general conditioning* with three sessions per week

1 week of full-body *hypertrophy* with three sessions per week

1 week of full-body *strength* with three sessions per week

1 week of full-body *general conditioning* with three sessions per week

1 week of full-body *hypertrophy* with three sessions per week

1 week of full-body *strength* with three sessions per week

WEEKS	1	2	3	4	5	6	7	8
Metabolic phase	■	■	■					
Hypertrophy phase				■				
Strength phase					■			
Hypertrophy phase						■		
Strength phase							■	
Metabolic phase								■

or

3 weeks of *general conditioning* with split routines on four days a week

2 weeks of *hypertrophy* with split routine on four days a week

2 weeks of *strength* with split routines on four days a week

1 week of *general conditioning* with split routine over four days a week

2 weeks of *hypertrophy* with split routine on four days a week

2 weeks of *strength* with split routines on four days a week

WEEKS

	1	2	3	4	5	6	7	8	9	10	11	12
Metabolic phase	■	■	■									
Hypertrophy phase				■	■							
Strength phase						■	■					
Metabolic phase								■				
Hypertrophy phase									■	■		
Strength phase											■	■

or again we can foresee split routines in the micro cycle by dividing the week into **days** of *hypertrophy* and days of *strength* and after 4-6 weeks introduce a week of discharge.

DAYS

	1	2	3	4	5	6	7
Metabolic phase	■						
Hypertrophy phase		■	■				
Strength phase				■	■		

Within each periodization, the **type of progression of the loads and the volume of work** is decided.

Ultimately, the increases in loads can be **constant** from week to week (or every two weeks) or **cycled** (every week we start with a weight lower than the last workout but with a weight greater than the initial one). In the latter case, we can identify increasing variations between one workout and another in a constant manner or with variations every week or every certain number of workouts. Some graphs will clarify the concept.

In the graph below we see a simple progression of the loads carried out every week or every mesocycle.

Volume

2000							
1900							
1800							
1700							
1600							
1500							
1400							
1300							
1200							
1100							
1000							
900							
800							
700							
600							
500							
0							
Sets x reps	3 x 10		3 x 10		3 x 10		3 x 10
Weight Kg	30		40		50		60
Volume	900		1200		1500		1800

SIMPLE PROGRESSION

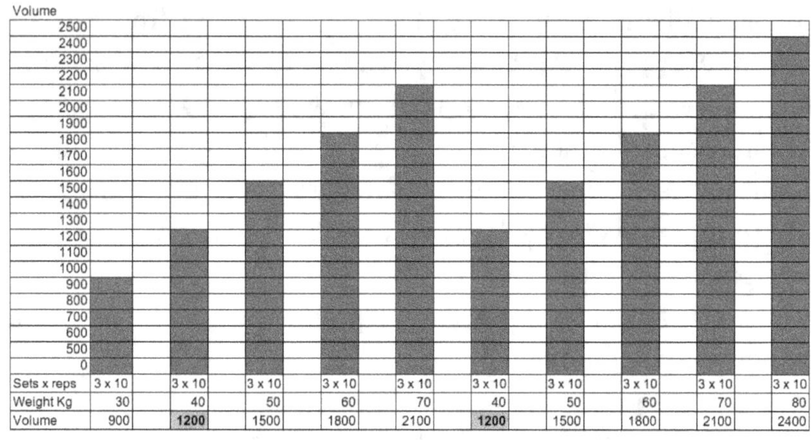

Sets x reps	3 x 10	3 x 10	3 x 10	3 x 10	3 x 10	3 x 10	3 x 10	3 x 10	3 x 10	3 x 10
Weight Kg	30	40	50	60	70	40	50	60	70	80
Volume	900	**1200**	1500	1800	2100	**1200**	1500	1800	2100	2400

STEP BACK

In this case, after a certain number of weeks in which the loads have progressively increased, lower loads are used again, starting however from a higher level than the initial level.

In our example, we start with a new cycle of increase using the weight lifted in the second week (40 kg.).

Implementing this type of load increase, leads to wave programming, as seen in the graph below.

Compared to a continuous linear increase, this modality allows a better phase of adaptation of the body to the efforts to which it is subjected while guaranteeing an increase in volume at the end of the macrocycle.

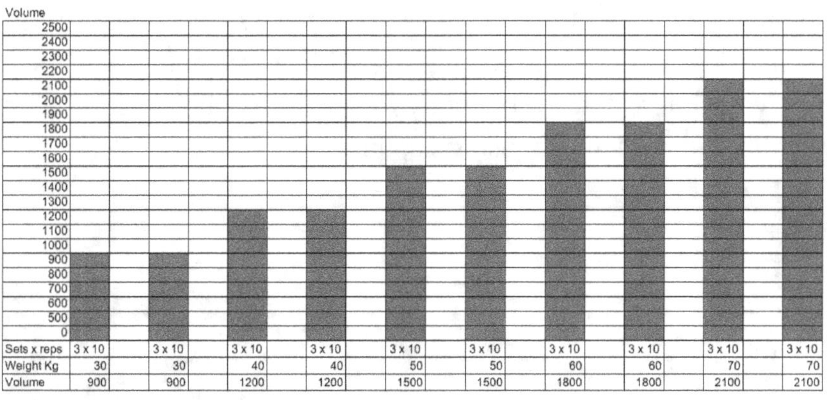

Sets x reps	3 x 10	3 x 10	3 x 10	3 x 10	3 x 10	3 x 10	3 x 10	3 x 10	3 x 10	3 x 10
Weight Kg	30	30	40	40	50	50	60	60	70	70
Volume	900	900	1200	1200	1500	1500	1800	1800	2100	2100

STEP

A further elaboration of this concept is given by the progression exemplified by the following graph, which describes a wave step back:

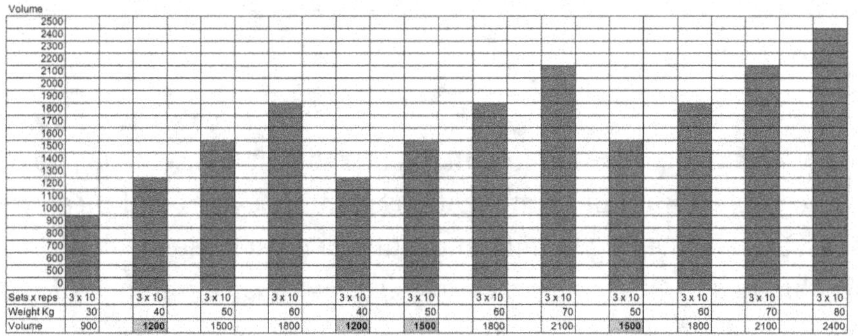

Sets x reps	3 x 10	3 x 10	3 x 10	3 x 10	3 x 10	3 x 10	3 x 10	3 x 10	3 x 10	3 x 10	3 x 10	3 x 10
Weight Kg	30	40	50	60	40	50	60	70	50	60	70	80
Volume	900	1200	1500	1800	1200	1500	1800	2100	1500	1800	2100	2400

WAVE

As can be deduced from the image, there are two phases of the progression of loads, which alternate from week to week.

A final example, called "steps", implies that the same load and volume is repeated for two consecutive weeks (or two consecutive mesocycles), before proceeding with increasing the load. In this way, time is left for the body to adapt to a given effort before pushing it to break homeostasis again.

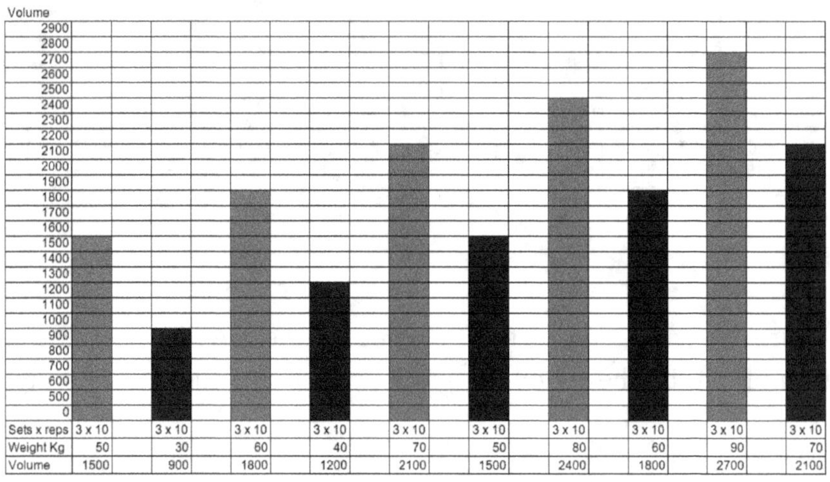

Sets x reps	3 x 10	3 x 10	3 x 10	3 x 10	3 x 10	3 x 10	3 x 10	3 x 10	3 x 10	3 x 10
Weight Kg	50	30	60	40	70	50	80	60	90	70
Volume	1500	900	1800	1200	2100	1500	2400	1800	2700	2100

WAVE STEP BACK

As you can see, keeping in mind the fixed points discussed above we can create infinite combinations in microcycles and mesocycles, always keeping in mind the individual response.

In this regard, it is necessary to **keep track** of the trends of the various sessions and then note the work done in terms of sets, repetitions, and load used, as well as the recovery time.

Below is an example of a page to keep track of workouts, which indicates the exercise performed, the number of repetitions, and the load used.

Workout Log Book

Date ....

WEIGHT	MON / TUE / WED / THU / FRI / SAT / SUN
MUSCLE GROUP	HOW I FEEL 1 / 2 / 3 / 4 / 5 / 6
START TIME	FINISH TIME

WATER

STRENGTH TRAINING

☐ UPPER BODY   ☐ LOWER BODY   ☐ ABS

CARDIO

EXERCISE	TIME	DISTANCE	CALS BURNED

EXERCISE	SET	1	2	3	4	5	6
	REPS						
	WEIGHT						
	REPS						
	WEIGHT						
	REPS						
	WEIGHT						
	REPS						
	WEIGHT						
	REPS						
	WEIGHT						
	REPS						
	WEIGHT						

To better understand how the body responds to training, it is also necessary to take note of some parameters such as **weight, temperature, circumferences, heart rate**. Find more information on measures and indices in my books dedicated to body recomposition such as "*Natural Bodybuilding and Body Recomposition - Slim with Muscles*" or "*Woman and Fitness*". For a whole year of training from which to take inspiration for your workouts and periodization I recommend my *"Complete 12 Months Workout Plan: Improve Fitness, Build Muscles, Increase Strenght"*.

Training Variables

Volume

The **volume** parameter represents the total amount of work done in a training session, or over a certain period. It is defined as the sum of the repetitions performed during the training session, or rather as the sum of the repetitions performed with a certain load: n.set * n.reps * Kg load.

The greater the volume, the heavier a training session for the same time.For example, 3 sets of 10 repetitions with 50kg are equal to 1500kg of volume. Adding up the volume done for each exercise of a given session will give you the total volume of the session.

Studies confirm that greater volume produces greater metabolic stress and greater hypertrophic response.

Therefore, by modifying one of the parameters of volume, its quantity is changed. If it is true that, assuming to lift 10 kg, the same volume is obtained with 10 sets of 10 repetitions or with 5 sets of 20 repetitions, at the level of muscle fatigue is not the same thing. Because with more sets is greater the possibility of muscle recovery (with the same rest time between one set and another) and the metabolism can rebuild the energy consumed in the movement of muscles.

Therefore, in addition to the load, the duration of the recovery times must also be considered.

The **load** is the other variable that constitutes the volume and is a variable directly related to hypertrophy, as practically all studies show, greater load corresponds to greater development.

To create our training plans, we already have these variables available: the number of sets, the duration of the rest between one set and another, the number of repetitions, and the load.

There is an inverse physical correlation between the lifted load and the number of repetitions: the higher the load, the lower the number of repetitions. It is a trivial and obvious equation for everyone. The load with which we can perform only one repetition, using a correct joint movement, is indicated with 1RM, representing the maximum limit, the load capacity of a given person. Below this limit and therefore with lower loads we can perform more than one repetition.

In general, scientific and practical evidence states that to train strength you must use loads of 80-90-100% of 1RM, to train hypertrophy loads of 65% to 80% of 1RM.

To train **strength**: 85%-100% 1RM
To train **hypertrophy**: 65%-85% 1RM

Frequency

The frequency parameter indicates how many times the training sessions are carried out, usually taking the week as a reference. We can also talk about training frequency for a single muscle group when evaluating how many times a particular muscle group has been trained.

The microcycle represents the period within which all muscle groups are trained. For convenience, the duration of a week is also taken as a reference. In this time frame, we can define training days and rest days between workouts. Research has shown that higher training frequencies lead, all other conditions being equal, to improvements in muscle mass. It is often discussed which is the best frequency, what is ultimately the recovery time needed between one session and another to maximize hypertrophy. In recent years, some research has been produced on this topic but there is still no precise scientific evidence on the optimal duration of recovery between one workout and another: some researchers conclude the need to allow at least 48 hours to pass between one session and another. Other researchers say it would be better to wait at least 72 hours. Usually, the more or less prefilled cards provide for 3 weekly workouts with one or more days of rest between workouts, especially in the case of **full-body** workouts. With this cadence, all the muscles of the body are trained at least three days a week. Or, for more advanced athletes, **split routines** are used in which not all muscle groups are trained in a single session but the muscles to be trained are separated, such as between muscles of the upper body and muscles of the lower body, being able in this way to increase the number of training sessions. A split routine allows also a greater variety of exercises for the trained muscles, for the same amount of time, compared to a routine that uses the full-body method. In any case, some authors highlight how resilience depends very much on the genetics of an individual. Again, several attempts and a greater scientific approach are needed to optimize efforts in terms of hypertrophy: not only affects the frequency with which you train but how you train, which muscles need more work because they tire less quickly, because they are mainly composed of slow-twitch fibers or because they have a greater recovery capacity.

Load (Intensity)

Load is one of the main variables that generate muscle hypertrophy. It defines the weight in kilograms raised during the repetitions.

It is a variable based on the level of training of the subject and his strength and to be used in the preparation of the various training protocols it must be understood in a relative sense, as a percentage of the maximum load lifted in a given exercise, as a percentage of the 1RM. Indirectly provides a measure of the intensity of the effort sustained during training.

The maximum repetition is indicated with "**1RM**". Researchers formulated some hypotheses concerning the value of the maximum repetition without having to establish it directly by testing. Tables have been compiled that relate the number of repetitions performed with a given load to establish the maximum load of a subject.

If, for example, a maximum of 10 repetitions are performed with 50kg, based on the table I have entered below, this corresponds to 75% of 1RM so the maximum load of this person in that particular exercise should be 67 kg. Beyond the formulas used, which may change over time with new research or studies, the table is convenient for our purposes to create personalized training workouts thus providing a starting point to record the progress of our efforts towards the desired goals.

Correlation
between maximum repetitions and intensity
as a percentage of 1RM

100% 1RM = 1 maximum repetition
95% 1RM = 2 maximum repetitions
93% 1RM = 3 maximum repetitions
90% 1RM = 4 maximum repetitions
87% 1RM = 5 maximum repetitions
85% 1RM = 6 maximum repetitions
83% 1RM = 7 maximum repetitions
80% 1RM = 8 maximum repetitions
77% 1RM = 9 maximum repetitions
75% 1RM = 10 maximum repetitions
70% 1RM = 11 maximum repetitions
67% 1RM = 12 maximum repetitions
65% 1RM = 15 maximum repetitions
60% 1RM = 20 maximum repetitions

Type of Exercises

Varying the exercises is essential for muscle development because it allows you to train different parts of the muscle, especially for those muscles that have different insertion points on the skeleton. If we take for example the deltoid or the trapezius or the pectoral, these have different insertions and conformations such that they are more activated by performing a given movement. For the pectoral group, for example, the central areas of that muscle will be stressed more with the flat bench, while with the inclined bench the upper areas will be stressed more. In general, an area of the muscle is affected differently according to the movement of a given exercise.

One of the main distinctions in the type of exercise is between **multi-joint** and **single-joint** exercises.

The former involves several muscle groups during their execution because the movement involves several joints at the same time, while the latter involves only one joint. Multiarticular exercises such as the squat are usually more demanding on a systemic level and can be used more in those phases where greater metabolic activation is required.

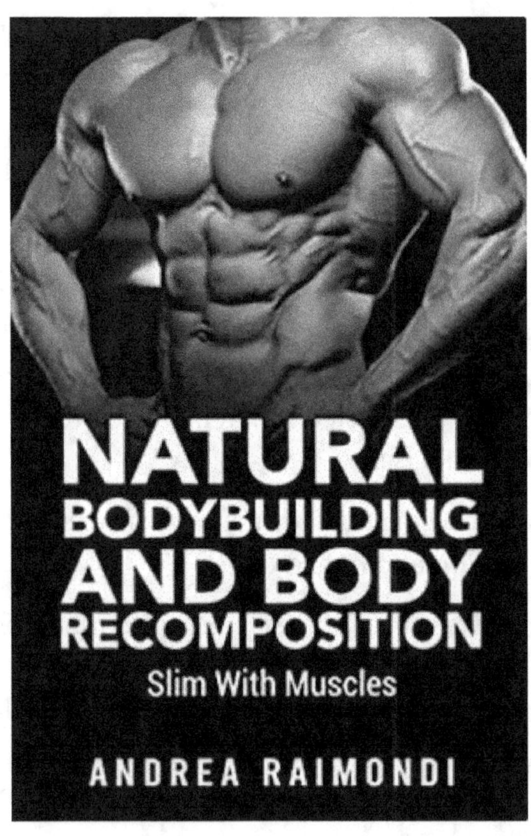
NATURAL
BODYBUILDING
AND BODY
RECOMPOSITION
Slim With Muscles
ANDREA RAIMONDI

Progression

Setting a progression in the training variables is essential to maximize the hypertrophic results of the training itself, always bearing in mind, however, that the right volume and load must be guaranteed during the training sessions. A progression concerns the change of one of the main training variables such as increasing the number of sets or repetitions or the load used between one microcycle and another or between one mesocycle and another.

For example, if in the first microcycle we held 3 sets for 12 repetitions using 15kg as maximum weight, in the following microcycle we can increase the sets, keeping the other parameters constant, so we will perform 5 sets for 12 repetitions with 15 kg, or we can increase the weight lift while holding the number of sets and reps, for example, we will do 3 sets for 12 reps with 17kg.

To check if you can maintain progression in your workouts, it is essential to keep a training diary in which we can write down exercises, loads, sets, repetitions, recovery times, and notes on the perception of effort. It will be possible to verify in practice whether our training is going in the desired direction.

TUT (Duration of Repetition)

TUT is the acronym for Time Under Tension, it indicates the duration of the muscle movement during a repetition. It is expressed in seconds.

If we think about the movement performed during a repetition, we notice that this can be broken down into 4 phases: a phase in which we move the weight by lifting it (called eccentric phase), a phase in which we reach maximum extension (or maximum contraction) and the movement stops (isometric stop) and then returns to the starting position by lowering the load (concentric phase), to finally stop the movement (isometric stop in shortened position) before starting the next repetition.

For each of these moments, it is possible to modify its duration: raising and lowering the load more slowly or faster, increasing or decreasing the duration of the pause between the two movements.

It is commonly used to express these four phases with figures such as 3141 which respectively indicate the duration in seconds of the eccentric phase, the duration of the stop in the extended position, the duration of the concentric phase, the duration of the stop in the shortened position.

Since there is no certain scientific evidence on the optimal time for the various phases of repetition, over time different schools of thought have been formed: there are those who affirm that it is the fast repetition that guarantees maximum muscle development and those who affirm the opposite, by aiming at a slow or very slow lift and return speed.

From our point of view, as for the other variables, it is necessary to experiment what is the best speed for a given person. In any case, it is essential to vary the stimuli in the various mesocycles from the point of view of the speed of execution also, keeping the only rule, to always keep a controlled movement and with execution as clean as possible, focusing on the muscle you are training.

We, therefore, have another arrow in our bow to try to stimulate muscle development and vary the stimuli to push the body to seek new homeostasis at a higher level than the previous one in terms of muscle mass.

Rest between Sets

Even with this training variable, it is possible to influence the results of muscle development because decreasing the pause time between one set and the next increases the metabolic stress and the hormonal and protein synthesis responses that we highlighted in the first chapter.

Therefore, with the same volume and intensity, minor pauses between sets lead to an accumulation of substances pro hypertrophy, but also a greater accumulation of fatigue.

The relationship between effort and fatigue must therefore be correctly measured. The experience in training and keeping track of the work done by noting the responses of one's body are highlighted using some physical parameters and some measurements, which we indicate in a subsequent chapter and can indicate the right mix between effort and fatigue for a given person.

Training Techniques

We present here some specific methodologies for resistance training developed over the years by practice in the gym.

There are no studies that demonstrate which methodology is the best over another, but even in this case, we can use these techniques as a tool that we can use to produce variability in training.

The fact remains that to obtain an increased muscle mass you need time, consistency, and a training plan that guarantees the correct increase in training stimuli.

CIRCUIT TRAINING

Circuit training involves the execution of a certain number of exercises, completing a setss for each exercise and moving on to the next without rest between one setss and another. At the end of the established exercises, rest is performed. At the end of rest time resumes with the first exercise foreseen in the training plan. Canceling the rest between one exercise and another increases cardiovascular work, increases metabolic stress and the aerobic phase. For these reasons it can be used in programs aimed at weight loss.

It can be used among others in the following ways:

• Organizing the entire training session in a single circuit to be repeated a set number of times.

• Setting the training session with 2 or more mini-circuits, perhaps divided by muscle areas.

PYRAMIDALS

Training with the pyramid method is based on the principle of providing an increase in the weight lifted with each set. The greater load and the fatigue that gradually accumulates in the trained muscle leads to a decrease in the number of repetitions.

For example:
1st set: 12 reps (50% 1RM)
2nd set: 10 repetitions (increasing kg)
3rd set: 8 repetitions (increasing kg)
4th set: 6 repetitions (increasing kg)
5th set: 4 repetitions (increasing kg)
You may continue with other sets by reducing the load and increasing the reps
6th set: 10 repetitions (decreases the kg)
7th set: 12 repetitions (decreases the kg)

DESCENDING PYRAMIDALS

In this case, we start with a high weight and we perform a few repetitions and with each repetition, we remove the weight and increase the repetitions.

For example:

1st set: 85% 1RM X 5 reps (or to muscle failure)
2nd set: 80% 1RM X 6 reps (or to muscle failure)
3rd set: 75% 1RM X 7 reps (or to muscle failure)
4th set: 70% 1RM X 9 reps (or to muscle failure)

BULGARIAN METHOD (heavy / light)

It consists of performing a set to exhaustion with a high load and a range of repetitions ranging from a minimum of four to a maximum of six; once concentric exhaustion is reached, the weight to be lifted will be unloaded by 20-30% and you will continue to push until muscular exhaustion.

It is important to minimize the dwell time between the two sets as if we were in theory carrying out a single set which includes unloading of the weight lifted.

The purpose of the first part of the sets, that is the heavy sets, is to recruit a large number of white fibers and try to bring them to exhaustion.

With the second part of the sets, the one carried out after unloading the weight, it will be possible to continue working the fibers not yet recruited, also leading to exhaustion.

For this purpose, the unloading of the weight from the tool is decisive, which must be such (from 20 to 30% of the initial load) as to allow the work to be continued for the necessary time, performing at least 6 to 8 repetitions, to exhaust the availability energy of the fibers involved.

REST PAUSE

With this technique, you perform a limited number of repetitions (6 or 8) with a high weight (90% 1RM).
Reached exhaustion, rest for 15-20 seconds and perform a repetition, another rest of 15-20 seconds and do another repetition, continuing for another three or more repetitions.

REPETITIONS 1 and 1/4

With this technique, one repetition is performed. At the end of the lifting phase, a second repetition is performed but not for the entire arc of the movement as usual but a partial arc (usually a quarter of the movement), repeating the procedure for the number of repetitions provided.

It is therefore a question of stopping in the final position of the movement and going back by ¼ of the movement and performing the partial repetition.

FORCED REPETITIONS

This is a method that involves the help of a training partner who, after muscle failure has been reached, helps to complete a certain number of other repetitions by lifting the weight.

21 (7 + 7 + 7)

This technique involves performing 21 consecutive repetitions for each set by dividing them into three different movements: 7 repetitions by lifting the load up to mid-movement, 7 repetitions with the full range of motion, and 7 repetitions from the intermediate to the final position of maximum contraction.

There may be different variations based on the moment in which the complete movement is performed, which can be performed at the beginning, in the middle, or at the end of the sets.

BULLDOZER SET

This method consists of completing a predetermined number of repetitions, usually from 30 to 50, stopping each time you reach muscle failure, and then resuming the sets until you reach the established number of repetitions. The longer the set goes on, the more rest must increase between one partial set and another.

INTERRUPTED SET

This method involves performing 5 repetitions with a weight equal to 80% 1RM and then rest for 20 seconds, perform another 5 repetitions with the same weight, rest another 20 seconds and perform other repetitions until failure. After a 3 minute break, do a new set.

SUPER SLOW

This method involves performing the repetitions in the slowest and most controlled way possible, for both the eccentric and concentric phases, for example, 10 seconds for the concentric phase and 5 seconds for the eccentric phase.

STRIPPING

With this technique, a certain number of repetitions are performed with a high load and the weight is gradually decreased by performing the maximum possible number of repetitions at each load change. For example, we start with 80% 1RM for 5-6 repetitions, unload the weight (10-15%), and when muscle exhaustion is reached, unload again and do repetitions until muscle exhaustion.

SUPERSET

It involves performing two exercises one after another, performing a set of one and a set of the other, and resting only at the end of the two sets. These are the main variants:

Superset for antagonist muscles. In this variant, the two exercises to be performed in superset refer to two antagonistic muscle groups, for example, Pectoral – Back or Biceps – Triceps or Quadriceps – Femoral.

Superset for same muscle group: The two exercises to be performed in superset refer to the same muscle group.

Usually, the superset consists of a basic multi-joint exercise and a secondary one which is usually an isolation exercise. A classic example would be for pectoral muscles: Barbell flat bench pushes + Dumbbell incline bench pushes. Or for the lats: Lat-machine tractions + Pulley.

TRISET

A technique similar to supersets, but the exercises to be performed are three, usually of the same muscle group. It allows great muscular exhaustion. This technique is usually used on large muscle groups that can support these types of work such as the pecs, lats, quadriceps.

=== Andrea Raimondi ===

Functional Evaluation

With functional evaluation, we can monitor the performance of a subject and then evaluate whether the program is progressing in the desired direction. As far as bodybuilding is concerned and to set the training schedules, some tests are important that allow you to know the **maximum** in a given exercise.

As we saw in another chapter, the training tables take into account the percentages of load compared to the maximum load in a given exercise. Furthermore, performing the tests at the end of each mesocycle can testify to the increase or decrease in strength of an athlete and therefore allows you to correct the variables of training or nutrition.

1RM Test

5 are performed by establishing which maximum weight it was possible to lift by the subject, increasing the weight with each lift.

Brzycki's formula

With this formula, the maximum of the subject can be obtained indirectly through the number of repetitions performed with a given load.

1 theoretical RM = lifted load / [1.0278 - (0.0278 x repetitions performed)]

This is just one of the many formulas proposed by the scientific literature for calculating the ceiling. From our point of view, it can be useful as an index of the subject's physical capacity.

Heart rate

This parameter can be useful for monitoring the state of fatigue and also for setting various training programs. Starting from the approximate calculation of the maximum heart rate given by 220 - age, we can derive the optimal heart rate percentages based on the goal you have:

For cardiovascular training, 70-80% of the HR Max

For weight loss 60-70% of the HR Max

For moderate activity, 50-60% of the HR Max

For a more precise calculation, the Karvonen formula can be used, which takes into account the resting heart rate. In this way, the reserve heart rate is obtained, which is multiplied by the percentage of work you want to keep and added to the resting heart rate provides the heart rate to keep during physical activity, as per the following formulas.

Reserve HR (HRres) = HRmax - Resting HR

relative intensity = HRres X % HRris + Resting HR

Aerobic activity

Aerobic activity is that type of motor activity that requires high consumption of oxygen as it lasts over time. As we have seen when talking about energy systems, the glycogen stores are depleted as a result of prolonged muscular work overtime; this leads to an increase in the use of energy reserves in the form of fats.

Aerobic activity is therefore useful in weight loss or in a phase of muscle definition, which can follow a so-called "mass" phase because it allows you to consume more calories than weight lifting. And obviously the longer the motor activity lasts over time, the higher the energy consumption will be. A moderate speed run is usually recommended, trying to keep your heart rate between 65 and 80% of your maximum heart rate.

This maximum heart rate can be obtained in a rough but indicative way with the following formula:

FCMax = 220 - age.

The minimum duration of aerobic activity recommended, to have a benefit over time in terms of physical condition and metabolic improvement, is at least 20 minutes per session.

In any case, you do not lose weight while doing the physical activity but maintaining a calorie deficit over time. Aerobic activity helps this process because it increases the consumption of calories and therefore allows the share of the aforementioned calorie deficit to be increased.

To get an idea of the role of aerobic activity in weight loss, we can use some useful formulas, developed over time by sports science scholars, such as the following:

Energy expenditure (Kcal) = 1Kcal x Kg of weight x Km traveled (Arcelli formula). For example 1Kcal x 60 (weight) x 10 (Km traveled) = 600 Kcal consumed.

Based on some studies, the percentages of use of carbohydrates and fats have been established as a function of the percentage of maximum heart rate, through the Respiratory Quotient and VO-max (oxygen consumption).

A heart rate below 80% of the maximum heart rate leads us to burn an average of 70% of carbohydrates and 30% of fat. Returning to our example, to know the amount of Kcal of fat burned we must calculate 30% of 600 Kcal, which corresponds to 180 Kcal. One gram of fat corresponds to 9 Kcal, but in the human body, the fat mass (adipocyte) is combined with water, for which 1Kg of body fat represents about 7,000 Kcal and not 9,000 Kcal, as it may seem by multiplying 1Kg by the 9 Kcal generated from a 1 gram of fat. So in practice, 1 gram of body fat corresponds to 7Kcal. In practice, in the training session of our example, 180 Kcal / 7 = 25.7 grams of fat were consumed. To lose, for example, 2.57 Kg. (25.7 grams * 1000 grams (1Kg)), keeping all other parameters unchanged, you have to travel 10,000 km. It is clear that to obtain results in terms of weight loss, one cannot ignore a diet that generates a long-term caloric deficit. And this is true regardless of the type of diet in vogue at any given time. You can also lose weight by eating more carbohydrates if your overall calorie intake is lower than your energy consumption.

Which aerobic activity to use? Much depends on personal preferences and the season. It is always preferable to carry out this activity outdoors, through running or jogging.

For those who start now with some aerobic activity, for example with running, I recommend starting with light activity, with 20-minute walks.

During the first phase, we will try to increase the duration of the training by 5-10 minutes at each outing, up to 45 minutes.

In the second phase, after the first 15 minutes of walking, a light run is started, to be held for 5 minutes. At this stage, we will try to increase the time in which we run each time, compared to the time in which we walk.

When you can run for at least 45 minutes, you can increase your running speed.

In this case, periods of slow running will alternate with periods of fast running.

For example, 15 minutes of slow running, 5 minutes of fast running, alternating between the two speeds during the training session, and trying each time to increase the duration of the fast run.

Phase 1 and phase 2 summary table for anaerobic training, in this case referring to running, of an untrained person. If you only practice aerobic activity, at least 3 workouts a week are recommended. If, on the other hand, you also practice weight training sessions, one or two sessions per week, depending on the type of preparation (whether for strength, mass, or general conditioning).

	PHASE 1	Time in minutes	
	WALK TIME	RUNNING TIME	TOTAL TIME
WEEK 1	20		20
WEEK 2	30		30
WEEK 3	40		40
WEEK 4	45		45

	PHASE 2	Time in minutes	
	WALK TIME	RUNNING TIME	TOTAL TIME
WEEK 1	15	10	25
WEEK 2	15	15	30
WEEK 3	15	20	35
WEEK 4	15	25	40

DEFINE GOALS

It is essential to be clear about the goal to be achieved. This is true in all human activities. Without having defined what you want to achieve from your training, it becomes difficult to correctly set up a program with the related exercise workouts.

The more precise the goal, the better it will be possible to calibrate the interventions based on the progress of the path as the program unfolds.

The main goals that you want to achieve with a scheduled workout can concern an **increase in muscle mass**, an **increase in strength**, a **decrease in body fat**. Although at first glance it may seem that the aforementioned goal are all linked to each other, this is not true in practice: there are different principles to be followed in the construction of plans aimed at achieving one or the other goal.

In all cases, however, it is necessary to establish a **starting point**. In our case, it concerns the **maximum weight** that can be lifted in a given exercise. For this, we must at least know directly or indirectly the maximum load from which the training progression will then derive. See the next paragraph for this. Furthermore, it is necessary to **keep track** of the results obtained in each training session, hence the need to keep a training **diary**, in paper or electronic form, as indicated in a previous chapter.

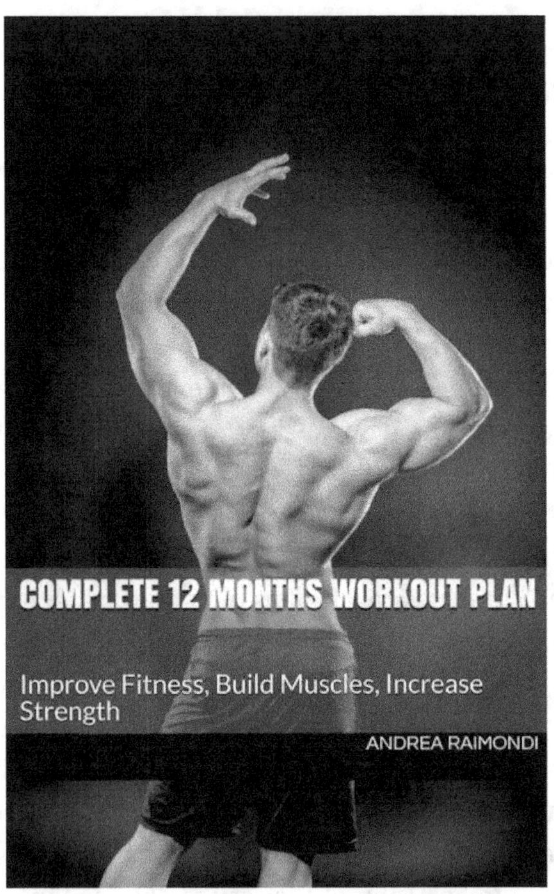
COMPLETE 12 MONTHS WORKOUT PLAN
Improve Fitness, Build Muscles, Increase Strength
ANDREA RAIMONDI

"This book gives you what most workout programs lack: a definite guide how to structure your weight lifting throughout a year's course. For a few bucks you get a solid template for a reasonable macrocycle. The exercise selection is pretty raw, nothing fancy at all - but then again Raimondi offers more of a fundamental template you can customize as you get more experience - not the next shiny new workout fad you see on social media these days. Beginners though can follow the plan simply as it is. Great prize value." Recensione di B. Lehner Amazon (versione inglese)

DEFINE THE PATH

We have previously seen the fundamental principles that distinguish the various goals, which I report here for convenience. This allows to build a progression that takes the form of a set of training sessions, in which the different training variables will vary. It is always good to insert an ***unloading phase after a cycle of strength or hypertrophy***. For weight loss, on the other hand, it is necessary to increase the metabolic work by reducing recovery times, by inserting aerobic work sessions in workouts. I have indicated a progression for aerobic activity in the chapter dedicated to it.

Metabolic phase or discharge
Series: 2/3
Reps: 20/25
Load: up to 60% 1RM

Hypertrophy phase
Series: 3/4
Reps: 6/12
Load: at 60% -80% 1RM

Strength phase
Series: 4/5
Reps: 3/5
Load: at 85% -100% 1RM

How long does a bulking phase last? And one of strength?

There are no fixed or scientifically established rules.

In general, for convenience, it is good to set up a macrocycle by dividing it into mesocycles of at least four weeks each, keeping some body measurements monitored that can indicate when the time has come to insert a discharge phase.

These measurements include *body temperature* and *heart rate* which are the main readings that indicate when the body begins to tire. So we can set for example 8 weeks of strength, with a progression in the loads as reported above. And enter a week of discharge after the first four weeks because we have detected a decreasing body temperature compared to the first weeks, or maybe this change occurs after the sixth or seventh week. Each body is different and responds differently to training stimuli, all other conditions being equal.

Concerning the **unloading phase**, it is possible to define a **partial**, **medium**, or **strong decrease** in training volume, based on the perceived level of fatigue. An unloading phase can last one or more weeks based on the measurements made.

A **partial unloading phase** may consist, for example, in reducing the work by just one series compared to a "normal" training session. Or you can reduce the load carried out by reducing the amount of perceived effort: if you worked with 80% of the maximum, use loads of 70% of the maximum for the same series and repetitions for the protocol followed.

An **average unloading phase** can consist in halving the series performed for a given exercise and reducing the loads used by 10-15%.

A **strong-type unloading phase** may consist in performing only isolation exercises for a given muscle district, performing 3 series for 12 repetitions with a load equal to 65% of the maximum load. Again there are no fixed rules but only individual practice and measurements can determine if we are moving in the right direction.

[66]

THE STEPS TO FOLLOW

Below are the steps to follow to create workouts inserted within the established schedule.

1) After determining our goal, we decide whether to follow a traditional **periodization** or a wavy periodization.

2) Find **maximal** for each exercise, directly or indirectly, as seen above.

3) **Training days** are determined for each week of the mesocycle

4) **Progression of the loads** is determined, in the case of a strength or hypertrophy protocol. It will be a question of defining the increase in the number of repetitions or the reduction of recovery times in cases of metabolic protocols.

5) Choose, for each mesocycle, the **type of split routine** or full-body sessions.

6) Choose the **technique** for each mesocycle and the single weekly session within the mesocycle: that is, choose whether to perform pyramids or supersets, etc ...

7) Choose **exercises** for each muscle district in each training session scheduled for a given mesocycle.

8) Finally, find the number of series, repetitions, TUT and rest time between the series based on the load initially determined for each planned exercise.

Below is a series of sample workouts based on the different protocols.
In all exercises a TUT of 2121 is used, therefore with slow and controlled execution.

Strength phase

Strength phase. Section 1. Week 1
Perceived effort level 8, increase the weight after each set, the last until muscle failure

DAY	MUSCLES	EXERCICES
Monday	Full Body	Bench press [3 sets @ 5-6 RM] Military press [3 sets @ 5-6 RM] Low pulley row [3 sets @ 5-6 RM] Dumbbell curl [3 sets @ 5-6 RM] Cable pushdown [3 sets @ 5-6 RM] Leg curl [3 sets @ 5-6 RM] Squat [3 sets @ 5-6 RM] Crunch [3 sets @ 15-20RM]
Tuesday	Rest	
Wednesday	Full Body	Bench press [3 sets @ 5-6 RM] Military press [3 sets @ 5-6 RM] Low pulley row [3 sets @ 5-6 RM] Dumbbell curl [3 sets @ 5-6 RM] Cable pushdown [3 sets @ 5-6 RM] Leg curl [3 sets @ 5-6 RM] Squat [3 sets @ 5-6 RM] Crunch [3 sets @ 15-20RM]
Thursday	Rest	
Friday	Full Body	Bench press [3 sets @ 5-6 RM] Military press [3 sets @ 5-6 RM] Low pulley row [3 sets @ 5-6 RM] Dumbbell curl [3 sets @ 5-6 RM] Cable pushdown [3 sets @ 5-6 RM] Leg curl [3 sets @ 5-6 RM] Squat [3 sets @ 5-6 RM] Crunch [3 sets @ 15-20RM]
Saturday	Rest	Aerobic Activity
Sunday	Rest	

Strength phase. Section 1. Week 2
Perceived effort level 8, increase the weight after each set, the last until muscle failure

DAY	MUSCLES	EXERCICES
Monday	Full Body	Bench press [3 sets @ 3-5 RM] Military press [3 sets @ 3-5 RM] Low pulley row [3 sets @ 3-5 RM] Dumbbell curl [3 sets @ 3-5 RM] Cable pushdown [3 sets @ 3-5 RM] Leg curl [3 sets @ 3-5 RM] Squat [3 sets @ 3-5 RM] Crunch [3 sets @ 15-20RM]
Tuesday	Rest	
Wednesday	Full Body	Bench press [3 sets @ 3-5 RM] Military press [3 sets @ 3-5 RM] Low pulley row [3 sets @ 3-5 RM] Dumbbell curl [3 sets @ 3-5 RM] Cable pushdown [3 sets @ 3-5 RM] Leg curl [3 sets @ 3-5 RM] Squat [3 sets @ 3-5 RM] Crunch [3 sets @ 15-20RM]
Thursday	Rest	
Friday	Full Body	Bench press [3 sets @ 3-5 RM] Military press [3 sets @ 3-5 RM] Low pulley row [3 sets @ 3-5 RM] Dumbbell curl [3 sets @ 3-5 RM] Cable pushdown [3 sets @ 3-5 RM] Leg curl [3 sets @ 3-5 RM] Squat [3 sets @ 3-5 RM] Crunch [3 sets @ 15-20RM]
Saturday	Rest	Aerobic Activity
Sunday	Rest	

Strength phase. Section 1. Week 3

Perceived effort level 8, increase the weight after each set, the last until muscle failure

DAY	MUSCLES	EXERCICES
Monday	Full Body	Bench press [3 sets @ 1-3 RM] Military press [3 sets @ 1-3 RM] Low pulley row [3 sets @ 1-3 RM] Dumbbell curl [3 sets @ 1-3 RM] Cable pushdown [3 sets @ 1-3 RM] Leg curl [3 sets @ 1-3 RM] Squat [3 sets @ 1-3 RM] Crunch [3 sets @ 15-20RM]
Tuesday	Rest	
Wednesday	Full Body	Bench press [3 sets @ 1-3 RM] Military press [3 sets @ 1-3 RM] Low pulley row [3 sets @ 1-3 RM] Dumbbell curl [3 sets @ 1-3 RM] Cable pushdown [3 sets @ 1-3 RM] Leg curl [3 sets @ 1-3 RM] Squat [3 sets @ 1-3 RM] Crunch [3 sets @ 15-20RM]
Thursday	Rest	
Friday	Full Body	Bench press [3 sets @ 1-3 RM] Military press [3 sets @ 1-3 RM] Low pulley row [3 sets @ 1-3 RM] Dumbbell curl [3 sets @ 1-3 RM] Cable pushdown [3 sets @ 1-3 RM] Leg curl [3 sets @ 1-3 RM] Squat [3 sets @ 1-3 RM] Crunch [3 sets @ 15-20RM]
Saturday	Rest	Aerobic Activity
Sunday	Rest	

Hypertrophy phase

Hypertrophy phase. Mesocycle 1. Week 1

DAY	MUSCLES	EXERCICES
Monday	Full Body	Dumbbell bench press [3 sets @ 10-12RM] Dumbbell military press [3 sets @ 10-12RM] Low pulley row [3 sets @ 10-12RM] Dumbbell curl [3 sets @ 10-12RM] Cable pushdown [3 sets @ 10-12RM] Leg curl [3 sets @ 10-12RM] Leg extension [3 sets @ 10-12RM] Crunch [3 sets @ 10-12RM] Calf raise [3 sets @ 10-12RM]
Tuesday	Rest	
Wednesday	Full Body	Dumbbell flyes [3 sets @ 10-12RM] Lateral raises [3 sets @ 10-12RM] Lat Machine [3 sets @ 10-12RM] Dumbbell curl [3 sets @ 10-12RM] Cable pushdown [3 sets @ 10-12RM] Leg curl [3 sets @ 10-12RM] Leg extension [3 sets @ 10-12RM] Crunch [3 sets @ 10-12RM] Calf raise [3 sets @ 10-12RM]
Thursday	Rest	
Friday	Full Body	Dumbbell bench press [3 sets @ 10-12RM] Dumbbell military press [3 sets @ 10-12RM] Low pulley row [3 sets @ 10-12RM] Dumbbell curl [3 sets @ 10-12RM] Cable pushdown [3 sets @ 10-12RM] Leg curl [3 sets @ 10-12RM] Leg extension [3 sets @ 10-12RM] Crunch [3 sets @ 10-12RM] Calf raise [3 sets @ 10-12RM]
Saturday	Rest	Aerobic Activity
Sunday	Rest	

Hypertrophy phase. Mesocycle 1. Week 2

DAY	MUSCLES	EXERCICES
Monday	Full Body	Dumbbell bench press [3 sets @ 8-10RM] Dumbbell military press [3 sets @ 1 8-10RM] Low pulley row [3 sets @ 8-10RM] Dumbbell curl [3 sets @ 8-10RM] Cable pushdown [3 sets @ 8-10RM] Leg curl [3 sets @ 8-10RM] Leg extension [3 sets @ 8-10RM] Crunch [3 sets @ 8-10RM] Calf raise [3 sets @ 8-10RM]
Tuesday	Rest	
Wednesday	Full Body	Dumbbell flyes [3 sets @ 8-10RM] Lateral raises [3 sets @ 8-10RM] Lat Machine [3 sets @ 8-10RM] Dumbbell curl [3 sets @ 8-10RM] Cable pushdown [3 sets @ 8-10RM] Leg curl [3 sets @ 8-10RM] Leg extension [3 sets @ 8-10RM] Crunch [3 sets @ 8-10RM] Calf raise [3 sets @ 8-10RM]
Thursday	Rest	
Friday	Full Body	Dumbbell bench press [3 sets @ 8-10RM] Dumbbell military press [3 sets @ 1 8-10RM] Low pulley row [3 sets @ 8-10RM] Dumbbell curl [3 sets @ 8-10RM] Cable pushdown [3 sets @ 8-10RM] Leg curl [3 sets @ 8-10RM] Leg extension [3 sets @ 8-10RM] Crunch [3 sets @ 8-10RM] Calf raise [3 sets @ 8-10RM]
Saturday	Rest	Aerobic Activity
Sunday	Rest	

Hypertrophy phase. Mesocycle 1. Week 3

Loads are increased and repetitions reduced, always with maximum control of movement. Recovery between one set and another of 60 secs..

DAY	MUSCLES	EXERCICES
Monday	Full Body	Dumbbell bench press [3 sets @ 6-8RM] Dumbbell military press [3 sets @ 6-8RM] Low pulley row [3 sets @ 6-8RM] Dumbbell curl [3 sets @ 6-8 RM] Cable pushdown [3 sets @ 6-8RM] Leg curl [3 sets @ 6-8RM] Leg extension [3 sets @ 6-8RM] Crunch [3 sets @ 6-8RM] Calf raise [3 sets @ 6-8RM]
Tuesday	Rest	
Wednesday	Full Body	Dumbbell flyes [3 sets @ 6-8RM] Lateral raises [3 sets @ 6-8RM] Lat Machine [3 sets @ 6-8RM] Dumbbell curl [3 sets @ 6-8RM] Cable pushdown [3 sets @ 6-8RM] Leg curl [3 sets @ 6-8RM] Leg extension [3 sets @ 6-8RM] Crunch [3 sets @ 6-8RM] Calf raise [3 sets @ 6-8RM]
Thursday	Rest	
Friday	Full Body	Dumbbell bench press [3 sets @ 6-8RM] Dumbbell military press [3 sets @ 6-8RM] Low pulley row [3 sets @ 6-8RM] Dumbbell curl [3 sets @ 6-8 RM] Cable pushdown [3 sets @ 6-8RM] Leg curl [3 sets @ 6-8RM] Leg extension [3 sets @ 6-8RM] Crunch [3 sets @ 6-8RM] Calf raise [3 sets @ 6-8RM]
Saturday	Rest	Aerobic Activity
Sunday	Rest	

Hypertrophy phase. Mesocycle 1. Week 4
Unloading week, before the new Mesocycle, decrease loads and increase repetitions, rest 45-60 "

DAY	MUSCLES	EXERCICES
Monday	Full Body	Dumbbell bench press [3 sets @ 10-12RM] Dumbbell military press [3 sets @ 10-12RM] Low pulley row [3 sets @ 10-12RM] Dumbbell curl [3 sets @ 10-12RM] Cable pushdown [3 sets @ 10-12RM] Leg curl [3 sets @ 10-12RM] Leg extension [3 sets @ 10-12RM] Crunch [3 sets @ 10-12RM] Calf raise [3 sets @ 10-12RM]
Tuesday	Rest	
Wednesday	Full Body	Dumbbell flyes [3 sets @ 10-12RM] Lateral raises [3 sets @ 10-12RM] Lat Machine [3 sets @ 10-12RM] Dumbbell curl [3 sets @ 10-12RM] Cable pushdown [3 sets @ 10-12RM] Leg curl [3 sets @ 10-12RM] Leg extension [3 sets @ 10-12RM] Crunch [3 sets @ 10-12RM] Calf raise [3 sets @ 10-12RM]
Thursday	Rest	
Friday	Full Body	Dumbbell bench press [3 sets @ 10-12RM] Dumbbell military press [3 sets @ 10-12RM] Low pulley row [3 sets @ 10-12RM] Dumbbell curl [3 sets @ 10-12RM] Cable pushdown [3 sets @ 10-12RM] Leg curl [3 sets @ 10-12RM] Leg extension [3 sets @ 10-12RM] Crunch [3 sets @ 10-12RM] Calf raise [3 sets @ 10-12RM]
Saturday	Rest	Aerobic Activity
Sunday	Rest	

In the two mesocycles just seen, the first for strength and the second for hypertrophy, we followed the dictates regarding the use of loads and the number of repetitions: the heavier the load to be lifted (relative to the strength of a given subject), the fewer repetitions you can lift. The strength protocol assumes that heavy loads are used, between 85% and 100% of the maximum repetition. In this case, therefore, the progression in the loads is highlighted by the fact that the repetitions, equal to the number of sets, decrease between one week and the next. The same happens in the protocol for hypertrophy but, in this case, we start from lower loads, between 60% and 80% of the maximum load (1RM).

In both protocols proposed, the week, or microcycle, includes three training sessions in full-body mode: all muscle groups are trained in each session.

If we combine the two protocols, strength and hypertrophy, within a macrocycle, we obtain a wavy periodization. In this case, it is good to insert at least one micro-cycle of discharge between the strength phase and the hypertrophy phase. The type of discharge, whether partial, medium, or strong, will depend, as seen, on the level of relative fatigue perceived at the end of the mesocycle. We will see shortly an example of the unloading phase. First I propose an example of a macrocycle of strength and hypertrophy using training sessions with split routines. Note: 6-8RM gives a measure of the load used. In this case, it is assumed that with the chosen load it is possible to perform a maximum of 8 repetitions and not less than 6. The more the repetitions increase, the lighter the weight used.

Strength Phase #2

Section 2. Week 1

DAY	MUSCLES	EXERCISES
Monday	Upper body	Bench Press [3 serie @ 6-8 RM] Military press [3 serie @ 6-8 RM] Dumbbells flyes [3 serie @ 6-8 RM] Lat machine [3 serie @ 6-8 RM] Dumbbells curl [3 serie @ 6-8 RM] Pull down [3 serie @ 6-8 RM]
Tuesday	Lower body	Leg curl [3 serie @ 6-8 RM] Squat [3 serie @ 6-8 RM] Calf raise [3 serie @ 6-8 RM] Crunch [3 serie @ 15-20RM]
Wednesday	Rest	
Thursday	Upper body	Bench Press [3 serie @ 6-8 RM] Military press [3 serie @ 6-8 RM] Dumbbell lateral raise [3 serie @ 6-8 RM] Lat machine [3 serie @ 6-8 RM] Dumbbells curl [3 serie @ 6-8 RM] Pull down [3 serie @ 6-8 RM]
Friday	Lower body	Leg curl [3 serie @ 6-8 RM] Squat [3 serie @ 6-8 RM] Calf raise [3 serie @ 6-8 RM] Crunch [3 serie @ 15-20RM]
Saturday	Rest	Aerobic Activity
Sunday	Rest	

Strength phase. Section 2. Week 2

DAY	MUSCLES	EXERCISES
Monday	Upper body	Bench Press [3 serie @ 3-5 RM] Military press [3 serie @ 3-5 RM] Dumbbells flyes [3 serie @ 3-5 RM] Lat machine [3 serie @ 3-5 RM] Dumbbells curl [3 serie @ 3-5 RM] Pull down [3 serie @ 3-5 RM]
Tuesday	Lower body	Leg curl [3 serie @ 3-5 RM] Squat [3 serie @ 3-5 RM] Calf raise [3 serie @ 3-5 RM] Crunch [3 serie @ 15-20RM]
Wednesday	Rest	
Thursday	Upper body	Bench Press [3 serie @ 3-5 RM] Military press [3 serie @ 3-5 RM] Dumbbell lateral raise [3 serie @3-5 RM] Lat machine [3 serie @ 3-5 RM] Dumbbells curl [3 serie @ 3-5 RM] Pull down [3 serie @ 3-5 RM]
Friday	Lower body	Leg curl [3 serie @ 3-5 RM] Squat [3 serie @ 3-5 RM] Calf raise [3 serie @ 3-5 RM] Crunch [3 serie @ 15-20RM]
Saturday	Rest	Aerobic Activity
Sunday	Rest	

Strength phase. Section 2. Week 3

DAY	MUSCLES	EXERCISES
Monday	Upper body	Bench Press [3 serie @ 2-3 RM] Military press [3 serie @ 2-3 RM] Dumbbells flyes [3 serie @ 2-3 RM] Lat machine [3 serie @ 2-3 RM] Dumbbells curl [3 serie @ 2-3 RM] Pull down [3 serie @ 2-3 RM]
Tuesday	Lower body	Leg curl [3 serie @ 2-3 RM] Squat [3 serie @ 2-3 RM] Calf raise [3 serie @ 2-3 RM] Crunch [3 serie @ 15-20RM]
Wednesday	Rest	
Thursday	Upper body	Bench Press [3 serie @ 2-3 RM] Military press [3 serie @ 2-3 RM] Dumbbell lateral raise [3 serie @2-3 RM] Lat machine [3 serie @ 2-3 RM] Dumbbells curl [3 serie @ 2-3 RM] Pull down [3 serie @ 2-3 RM]
Friday	Lower body	Leg curl [3 serie @ 2-3 RM] Squat [3 serie @ 2-3 RM] Calf raise [3 serie @ 2-3 RM] Crunch [3 serie @ 15-20RM]
Saturday	Rest	Aerobic Activity
Sunday	Rest	

In this new phase of strength, there are four training sessions, dividing the muscular districts into Upper body and Lower body split routines and maintaining three training series per exercise. Increasing the loads from one week to the next, as can be seen from the decrease in the number of repetitions for each exercise.

Hypertrophy Phase #2

Mesocycle 2. Week 1.

DAY	MUSCLES	EXERCISES
Monday	Chest, back, legs, abs	Dumbbells Bench Press [4 serie @ 10-12RM] Dumbbells flyes [4 serie @ 10-12RM] Pulley [4 serie @ 10-12RM] Leg curl [4 serie @ 10-12RM] Crunch [4 serie @ 10-12RM]
Tuesday	Shoulders, Legs, Abs	Military press [4 serie @ 10-12RM] Dumbbell lateral raise [4 serie @ 10-12RM] Dunmbbell rear raise [4 serie @ 10-12RM] Leg extension [4 serie @ 10-12RM] Leg Press [4 serie @ 10-12RM] Calf[4 serie @ 10-12RM] Crunch [4 serie @ 10-12RM]
Wednesday	Arms, Abs	Dumbbells curl [3 serie @ 10-12RM] Pull down [3 serie @ 10-12RM] Crunch [4 serie @ 10-12RM]
Thursday	Chest, back, legs, abs	Dumbbells Bench Press [4 serie @ 10-12RM] Dumbbells flyes [4 serie @ 10-12RM] Lat Machine [4 serie @ 10-12RM] Leg curl [4 serie @ 10-12RM] Crunch [4 serie @ 10-12RM]
Friday	Shoulders, Legs, Abs	Military press [4 serie @ 10-12RM] Dumbbell lateral raise [4 serie @ 10-12RM] Dumbbells rear raise [4 serie @ 10-12RM] Leg extension [4 serie @ 10-12RM] Leg Press [4 serie @ 10-12RM] Calf [4 serie @ 10-12RM] Crunch [4 serie @ 10-12RM]
Saturday	Rest	Aerobic Activity
Sunday	Rest	

Hypertrophy Phase. Mesocycle 2. Week 2.
The loads are increased, Rest 60-90 "

DAY	MUSCLES	EXERCISES
Monday	Chest, back, legs, abs	Dumbbells Bench Press [4 serie @ 8-10RM] Dumbbells flyes [4 serie @ 8-10RM] Pulley [4 serie @ 8-10RM] Leg curl [4 serie @ 8-10RM] Crunch [4 serie @ 15-20RM]
Tuesday	Shoulders, Legs, Abs	Military press [4 serie @ 8-10RM] Dumbbell lateral raise [4 serie @ 8-10RM] Dumbbells rear raise [4 serie @ 8-10RM] Leg extension [4 serie @ 8-10RM] Leg Press [4 serie @ 8-10RM] Calf[4 serie @ 8-10RM] Crunch [4 serie @ 15-20RM]
Wednesday	Arms, Abs	Dumbbells curl [4 serie @ 8-10RM] Pull down [4 serie @ 8-10RM] Crunch [4 serie @ 8-10RM]
Thursday	Chest, back, legs, abs	Dumbbells Bench Press [4 serie @ 8-10RM] Dumbbells flyes [4 serie @ 8-10RM] Lat Machine [4 serie @ 8-10RM] Leg curl [4 serie @ 8-10RM] Crunch [4 serie @ 15-20RM]
Friday	Shoulders, Legs, Abs	Military press [4 serie @ 8-10RM] Dumbbell lateral raise [4 serie @ 8-10RM] Dumbbells rear raise [4 serie @ 8-10RM] Leg extension [4 serie @ 8-10RM] Leg Press [4 serie @ 8-10RM] Calf [4 serie @ 8-10RM] Crunch [4 serie @ 15-20RM]
Saturday	Rest	Aerobic Activity
Sunday	Rest	

Hypertrophy Phase. Mesocycle 2. Week 3.
The number of series is increased with a medium-high load, Rest of 60-90 " between the series.

DAY	MUSCLES	EXERCISES
Monday	Chest, back, legs, abs	Dumbbells Bench Press [5 serie @ 8-10 RM] Dumbbells flyes [5 serie @ 8-10 RM] Pulley [5 serie @ 8-10 RM] Leg curl [5 serie @ 8-10 RM] Crunch [4 serie @ 15-20 RM]
Tuesday	Shoulders, Legs, Abs	Military press [5 serie @ 8-10 RM] Dumbbell lateral raise [5 serie @ 8-10 RM] Dumbbells rear raise [5 serie @ 8-10 RM] Leg extension [5 serie @ 8-10 RM] Leg Press [4 serie @ 8-10RM] Calf [5 serie @ 8-10 RM] Crunch [4 serie @ 15-20RM]
Wednesday	Arms, Abs	Dumbbells curl [5 serie @ 8-10RM] Pull down [5 serie @ 8-10RM] Crunch [4 serie @ 15-20RM]
Thursday	Chest, back, legs, abs	Dumbbells Bench Press [5 serie @ 8-10 RM] Dumbbells flyes [5 serie @ 8-10 RM] Lat Machine [5 serie @ 8-10 RM] Leg curl [5 serie @ 8-10 RM] Crunch [4 serie @ 15-20 RM]
Friday	Shoulders, Legs, Abs	Military press [5 serie @ 8-10 RM] Dumbbell lateral raise [5 serie @ 8-10 RM] Dumbbells rear raise [5 serie @ 8-10 RM] Leg extension [5 serie @ 8-10 RM] Leg Press [4 serie @ 8-10RM] Calf [5 serie @ 8-10 RM] Crunch [4 serie @ 15-20RM]
Saturday	Rest	Aerobic Activity
Sunday	Rest	

In the mesocycle just seen, the training sessions are five per week, using a split routine that emphasizes the development of the lower body muscles: exercises for legs (and abs) are performed in four out of five sessions. This is to highlight how, for example, in a split "Raimondi" the work on the deficient muscles, the legs, in this case, can be inserted. While the other muscle groups are trained twice a week.

The progression on the loads is the same seen in the previous hypertrophy phase, with the difference that the number of training series increased, passing from three to four for the first two weeks. In the third week, the sets went from four to five, keeping the same load lifted (8-10RM).

I have included this change to show how we can act not only on the weight variable but also on the number of series to increase the volume of a workout.

In all of these examples, rest is 60-90 seconds.

Setting a metabolic phase aimed at weight loss, in which it is important to raise the pace of training, the rest times will be reduced between one series and the next, perhaps by adopting circuit training techniques or using supersets or giant sets.

It is possible to combine the various phases, the various mesocycles proposed so far to build a macrocycle that contains phases of strength and hypertrophy suitable for those who train in terms of bodybuilding. On the other hand, those who have a primary interest in the development of force can alternate the two mesocycles of force. However, I recommend to check your state of fitness, through the measurement of body temperature and heart rate, to determine when to insert a discharge phase. In any case, it is advisable to insert this unloading phase after 5-6 weeks of training to prevent any situations of fatigue.

Example of a Full body session with **Giant Set**, in two AB sessions to be repeated for four weekly workout according to the ABAB scheme: perform one exercise after another, with loads that allow you to perform a maximum of 15 repetitions for a total of 6 series (in this form). Rest of two minutes between sets

A

MUSCLES	EXERCISES
Full Body Giant Set 6 series	Dumbbell lateral raise [@ 15RM] Dumbbell Flys [@ 15RM] French Press [@ 15RM] Lat Machine [@ 15RM] Hammer Curl [@ 15RM] Leg Press [@ 15RM]

B

MUSCLES	EXERCISES
Full Body Giant Set 6 series	Dumbbell Row [@ 15RM] Bench Press [@ 15RM] Military Press [@ 15RM] Curl EZ Bar [@ 15RM] Leg Press [@ 15RM]

Below is another micro-cycle in two full-body A-B sessions, to be repeated for four weekly sessions, with scheme A-B-A-B. In this case, for session A we have inserted a **super series** for the Lower Body. In session B the super series concerns the exercises for the upper body.

A

MUSCLES	EXERCISES
Full Body Upper body High Weight	Dumbbells Row [4 series @ 6-8RM] Rest 1 minute and 30 seconds Bench Press [4 series @ 6-8RM] Rest 1 minute and 30 seconds Military press [4 series @ 6-8RM] Rest 1 minute and 30 seconds
Lower body Low Weight	Super Set [4 series]: Leg Curl [@ 15RM] Leg Extension [@ 15RM] Rest 40 seconds Lunge [30 reps]

B

MUSCLES	EXERCISES
Full Body Lower body High Weight	Squat [4 series @ 6-8RM] Rest 1 minute and 30 seconds Deadlift [4 series @ 6-8RM] Rest 1 minute and 30 seconds
Upper body Low Weight	Super Set [4 series]: Dumbbells curl [@ 15RM] Dumbbell lateral raise [@ 15RM] Rest 40 seconds Super Set [4 serie]: Lat Machine [@ 15RM] Pectoral Machine [@ 15RM] Rest 40 seconds

RECOVERY PHASE

In this mesocycle we increase the reps by decreasing the maximum loads used. This gives the body the time it needs to recover after the strength phase, which was a period of intense work.

At the same time, we reduce the recovery time between one set and another to increase metabolic work.

This procedure can also be used in protocols for definition or weight loss in combination with a low-calorie diet.

As you will see, these are full-body sessions with loads that allow from 15 to 20 repetitions, therefore relatively low.

Also for the recovery phases, it is possible to use sessions with split routines for four or five weekly sessions.

What matters is to use loads that allow a high number of repetitions.

Recovery phase. Section 1. Week 1
Perceived effort equal to 6

DAY	MUSCLES	EXERCICES
Monday	Full Body	Dumbbell bench press [3 sets @ 15-20RM] Dumbbell military press [3 sets @ 15-20RM] Dumbbell bent over row [3 sets @ 15-20RM] Dumbbell curl [3 sets @ 15-20RM] Cable pushdown [3 sets @ 15-20RM] Leg curl [3 sets @ 15-20RM] Squat [3 sets @ 15-20RM] Crunch [3 sets @ 15-20RM] Calf raise [3 sets @ 15-20RM]
Tuesday	Rest	
Wednesday	Full Body	Dumbbell bench press [3 sets @ 15-20RM] Dumbbell military press [3 sets @ 15-20RM] Dumbbell bent over row [3 serie @15-20RM] Dumbbell curl [3 sets @ 15-20RM] Cable pushdown [3 sets @ 15-20RM] Leg curl [3 sets @ 15-20RM] Squat [3 sets @ 15-20RM] Crunch [3 sets @ 15-20RM] Calf raise [3 sets @ 15-20RM]
Thursday	Rest	
Friday	Full Body	Dumbbell bench press [3 sets @ 15-20RM] Dumbbell military press [3 sets @ 15-20RM] Dumbbell bent over row [3 sets @ 15-20RM] Dumbbell curl [3 sets @ 15-20RM] Cable pushdown [3 sets @ 15-20RM] Leg curl [3 sets @ 15-20RM] Squat [3 sets @ 15-20RM] Crunch [3 sets @ 15-20RM] Calf raise [3 sets @ 15-20RM]
Saturday	Rest	Aerobic Activity
Sunday	Rest	

Recovery phase. Section 1. Week 2
Perceived effort level 7

DAY	MUSCLES	EXERCICES
Monday	Full Body	Dumbbell bench press [3 sets @ 15-20RM] Dumbbell military press [3 sets @ 15-20RM] Dumbbell bent over row [3 sets @ 15-20RM] Dumbbell curl [3 sets @ 15-20RM] Cable pushdown [3 sets @ 15-20RM] Leg curl [3 sets @ 15-20RM] Squat [3 sets @ 15-20RM] Crunch [3 sets @ 15-20RM] Calf raise [3 sets @ 15-20RM]
Tuesday	Rest	
Wednesday	Full Body	Dumbbell bench press [3 sets @ 15-20RM] Dumbbell military press [3 sets @ 15-20RM] Dumbbell bent over row [3 sets @ 15-20RM] Dumbbell curl [3 sets @ 15-20RM] Cable pushdown [3 sets @ 15-20RM] Leg curl [3 sets @ 15-20RM] Squat [3 sets @ 15-20RM] Crunch [3 sets @ 15-20RM] Calf raise [3 sets @ 15-20RM]
Thursday	Rest	
Friday	Full Body	Dumbbell bench press [3 sets @ 15-20RM] Dumbbell military press [3 sets @ 15-20RM] Dumbbell bent over row [3 sets @ 15-20RM] Dumbbell curl [3 sets @ 15-20RM] Cable pushdown [3 sets @ 15-20RM] Leg curl [3 sets @ 15-20RM] Squat [3 sets @ 15-20RM] Crunch [3 sets @ 15-20RM] Calf raise [3 sets @ 15-20RM]
Saturday	Rest	Aerobic Activity
Sunday	Rest	

Recovery phase. Section 1. Week 3
Perceived effort level 8

DAY	MUSCLES	EXERCICES
Monday	Full Body	Dumbbell bench press [3 sets @ 15-20RM] Dumbbell military press [3 sets @ 15-20RM] Dumbbell bent over row [3 sets @ 15-20RM] Dumbbell curl [3 sets @ 15-20RM] Cable pushdown [3 sets @ 15-20RM] Leg curl [3 sets @ 15-20RM] Squat [3 sets @ 15-20RM] Crunch [3 sets @ 15-20RM] Calf raise [3 sets @ 15-20RM]
Tuesday	Rest	
Wednesday	Full Body	Dumbbell bench press [3 sets @ 15-20RM] Dumbbell military press [3 sets @ 15-20RM] Dumbbell bent over row [3 sets @ 15-20RM] Dumbbell curl [3 sets @ 15-20RM] Cable pushdown [3 sets @ 15-20RM] Leg curl [3 sets @ 15-20RM] Squat [3 sets @ 15-20RM] Crunch [3 sets @ 15-20RM] Calf raise [3 sets @ 15-20RM]
Thursday	Rest	
Friday	Full Body	Dumbbell bench press [3 sets @ 15-20RM] Dumbbell military press [3 sets @ 15-20RM] Dumbbell bent over row [3 sets @ 15-20RM] Dumbbell curl [3 sets @ 15-20RM] Cable pushdown [3 sets @ 15-20RM] Leg curl [3 sets @ 15-20RM] Squat [3 sets @ 15-20RM] Crunch [3 sets @ 15-20RM] Calf raise [3 sets @ 15-20RM]
Saturday	Rest	Aerobic Activity
Sunday	Rest	

WHICH EXERCISES TO USE

The classic distinction between multi-joint and single-joint exercises often generates confusion and stances that sometimes border on the grotesque. If used correctly, that is with a controlled movement and, inserted in mesocycles and macrocycles based on the notions we have explained so far, all the exercises lead to the achievement of planned goals. The muscle reacts to the stimulus it is subjected to.

Of course, if the goal is to increase metabolic work, perhaps to lose fat mass, the more muscles are involved, the greater the energy expenditure. In this case, it may make sense to use multi-joint exercises to a greater extent.

In a work aimed at hypertrophy, little changes. The muscle must be subjected to work that breaks the homeostasis to which the body tends, through an increased training load. For this purpose any kind of exercise is fine.

The same applies to the diatribe on *free weight* exercises (with dumbbells or barbells) or with machines found in the gym: the important thing is to subject the muscle to a training effort that forces the muscle to grow.

Therefore, from my point of view, the use of one exercise rather than another for a given muscle district becomes more a matter of personal taste than a dogmatic or scientific indication.

Below I propose a series of exercises, for each muscle district, which for me are to be preferred. But, I repeat, this is not an absolute law. What matters is correct execution, with a controlled movement that lasts the right amount of time. I leave it to the reader to interpret what the "right" time is. Every human body is different, the structure of the muscles differs from individual to individual, the number of types I and type II fibers differs from individual to individual and from muscle to muscle. Only by trying and verifying the results obtained is it possible to find and organize the optimal training.

CHEST
- Push-up
- Chest press
- Dumbbells bench press
- Inclined Dumbbells Bench Press
- Dumbbells flyes

DORSALS
- Pull Up
- Pulley
- Lat machine (narrow grip, wide grip)
- Pulley

SHOULDERS
- Slow forward dumbbells
- Dumbbell lateral raise
- Dumbbell Rear raises

BICEPS
- Dumbbells curl
- Barbell curl

TRICEPS
- Dumbbells French press
- Dumbbells Kick back
- Push down

LEGS
- Squat
- Lunge
- Leg press
- Leg extension
- Leg curl

ABDOMINAL MUSCLES
- Crunch
- Sit-ups
- Reverse Crunch

=== Andrea Raimondi ===

Lockdown

In this book, it is assumed that the gyms are open so exercises with some typical gym machines are proposed.

In periods of lockdown, we can replace most of the exercises with some equipment that we can use, or already have, at home: a basic set includes a bench, one or more sets of dumbbells, a pull-up bar.

All items can be easily purchased new or used. The most important thing is to have enough loads to stimulate muscle growth.

It is possible to replace the lack of adequate weight with an increase in the number of repetitions. This guarantees improvements especially for those not looking for increase strength.

To increase strength, weights must push the muscle to adapt its capacity and structure to the weight lifted, so it's important to have more loads.

The rule: little movement is better than no movement.

More complex is the work to be done outside the gym related to the legs in which we have to replace the machines such as presses, leg extensions, and leg curls with squats and lunges, increasing the number of repetitions and using the dumbbells here too.

If we really can't get any tools we can perform free body exercises such as push-ups, crunches, squats, lunges, and all their infinite variations that allow us at least to keep fit.

In this case, I advise you to adopt a plan that involves performing 50 push-ups per day, 50 bodyweight squats, and 50 crunches and increase the number up to 100 repetitions, divided into sets of 20, 25. With half an hour a day, you will feel like a tiger!

If you are not trained enough, set yourself the goal of reaching that level after one or two months, starting from where you are and increasing by 10 repetitions every day or every week, according to your starting form.

The secret lies in the willingness to perform one, two, three more repetitions every time you train: the muscles tone up making them work, they are made for that, and in the meantime increases the metabolism and energy consumption.

BIBLIOGRAPHY

Arienti, Giuseppe, Le basi molecolari della nutrizione, 3.Ed., Padova, Piccin, 2011

Delavier Frederic., The Strength Training Anatomy, Human Kinetic,(2011)

Esposito, Daniele, Project Diet 1 e 2, Milano, Project Invictus (2017)

Esquerdo, Óscar Maria Enciclopedia degli EXERCISES di muscolazione, Cesena, Elika srl Editrice (2011) Ed.Or. (2008)

Ferlito, Alessio Project Strength, Brescia, Project Invictus (2016)

Johnston, Brian D., Eccellenza Tecnica, Firenze, Sandro Ciccarelli Editore, (2007), Ed.Or. (2003)

Johnston, Brian D., La scienza dell'esercizio, Firenze, Sandro Ciccarelli Editore, (2006), Ed.Or. (2003)

Lafay, Olivier Il Metodo Lafay , Milano, L'Ippocampo, (2011)Ed.Or., Paris (2004)

Liparoti, Fabrizio Project bodybuilding, Brescia, Project Invictus (2018)

Lyle McDonald Ultimate Diet 2.0

McArdle, Katch, Katch Exercise Physiology (1994)

Neri M.,Bargossi A.,Paoli A Alimentazione fitness e salute, Cesena, Elika, (2002)

Roncari, Andrea Project Exercise vol 1 e 2, Milano, Project Invictus (2017-2018)

Schoenfeld, Brad Scienza e sviluppo dell'ipertrofia muscolare, Firenze (2017) Tit.Or.: Science and development of muscle hypertrophy (2016)

Schoenfeld, Brad M.A.X. Muscle Plan, Firenze, Olympian's (2019) Tit. or. The M.A.X. Muscle Plan (2013)

Schwarzenegger, Arnold, The new Encyclopedia of Modern Bodybuilding, New York (1998)
Weineck Jurgen, L'allenamento ottimale, Perugia,2.ed. (2009), Tit.or. Optimales Training, 15.Ed. (2007)
Weider Joe, Ultimate Bodybuilding (1988)

©2021 Andrea Raimondi
www.fitnessedintorni.it

AREdit.com

Contacts: info@aredit.com